Traditional Chiropractic:

A Layperson's Guide to How it Works &
Why it's Attacked

Dr. John Reizer

Dedication

*This book is dedicated to my colleagues – the ones willing to stand up for our profession.
You know who you are.*

Disclaimer

The information contained within this book has not been evaluated by the FDA. The information is for educational purposes only and is not intended to diagnose, treat, cure, or prevent any disease!

In addition, the information that has been written in this book is based upon the opinions of Dr. John Reizer. The information is not intended to replace a professional relationship between a patient and a healthcare specialist nor is it intended as medical advice. This information is provided solely for the purpose of sharing knowledge derived from the experience of Dr. John Reizer. The author strongly encourages readers to make healthcare decisions based upon their own independent research.

About the Author

Dr. John Reizer lives in Spartanburg, South Carolina with his wife and daughter. He has been a practicing chiropractor for over 32 years.

John has published numerous books on the subject of chiropractic. Additional information is available at www.johnreizer.com.

Introduction

In 2002, I co-authored my first chiropractic book that was dedicated to helping future practitioners open and properly operate a successful practice. I decided to take on such a project because I believed it was important to help young chiropractors become successful. New chiropractors are the lifeblood of our profession, and we need as many practicing doctors as possible if we are going to survive as a healthcare discipline in such a medically oriented society.

Nine years later, I am still trying to help chiropractors become successful in their private practices while simultaneously attempting to teach laypersons the value of a chiropractic adjustment. Whether the mode of communication has been through email, telephone, face to face conversations, or the many books that I've written, quite a few people have heard or read my advice regarding the subject of chiropractic.

As a former associate professor at a chiropractic college, I have had an opportunity to view the chiropractic profession from a different perspective than most of my colleagues. Because of this fact, I feel qualified to make certain comments, regarding the profession, which other doctors might hesitate to speak about.

Unlike most of my previous books, this text has been written for laypersons. The information that follows will help healthcare consumers understand the basics about traditional chiropractic.

Some of the subjects I have written about in this book might annoy certain individuals. One of the important things I have learned, during my career as a healthcare provider, is that many people in society are emotionally tied to their perceptions or how they view the world. When a person is emotionally vested in a specific point of view, it is often difficult to teach that individual an alternative concept. Some people walk through life under the illusion that they are open-minded about certain subjects, yet their emotional ties to a specific belief system often preclude them from embracing new concepts with objectivity.

In order to understand the true benefits of chiropractic care and why the powers that be (the medical industrial complex) continue to attack the profession's practice objectives; it is necessary to give readers a brief history lesson about the chiropractic profession.

As you will find out from reading this book, chiropractic has been under attack for a long time and when one fully understands the logic behind the profession's objective, it should become quite evident to readers why certain special interest groups, within the healthcare industry, want to destroy or redefine the profession.

In the eyes of certain organizations, chiropractic represents a major threat to the traditional healthcare model. Many medically funded organizations have made it a top priority to try and silence chiropractic's voice of common sense in an otherwise insane industry.

I have always believed that the beauty of chiropractic rests within the profession's practice objective. The objective is so simple to understand that even a young child could comprehend how it works with the controlling laws of nature.

After reading this book, I am hopeful that your understanding of healthcare will change. If I am able to help some members of society see a clearer picture of what is really happening in the modern healthcare arena, I will have accomplished one of my very personal life goals!

-Dr. John Reizer

The History of Chiropractic

The word chiropractic comes from the two Greek words *cheiro* and *praktos* which translated into English means the practice done with the hands. Throughout history, human beings have been experimenting with the art of spinal adjusting. There are many references found in ancient records giving accounts of this type of health methodology, which was used in an effort to promote healing in the sick and elderly.

Evidence of spinal adjusting has been found in documents that date back to ancient civilizations such as those found in China, Egypt, and Greece. This information was passed on in secret writings and eventually found its way to the 19th century where health practitioners discovered the same important connections between the nervous system, spinal integrity, and general health disorders.

Later on, an interest in spinal adjustments developed in many additional areas of the world, including America. Medical doctors began to regularly utilize such techniques on patients.

In 1895, Daniel David Palmer, a magnetic healer residing in Davenport, Iowa who was very knowledgeable in human anatomy and physiology, delivered the first modern day chiropractic adjustment to a deaf janitor named Harvey Lillard. The adjustment became famous as Mr. Lillard regained most of his hearing. At first, Palmer thought that he had accidentally stumbled on a cure for deafness. This, however, he found not to be the case as other patients with deafness did not respond in the same way as Mr. Lillard. Although this was somewhat frustrating, Palmer was not completely discouraged because in his failure to find a cure for deafness, he began to notice other physiological problems begin to improve in patients to whom he was administering chiropractic adjustments.

Palmer began to slowly make the connection that vertebrae which were out of their proper alignment were not causing a specific malady in the body, but instead were interfering with the body's natural abilities to process information from the brain. The brain was sending the proper messages for the body to be healthy. The misalignments in the spinal column were distorting these messages and the chemistry of the body began to make mistakes which eventually caused a decline in the health of that person. Palmer rationalized that a correction of these spinal misalignments would restore proper communication between brain and body, thus the biochemistry in the individual would balance out naturally.

Dr. Palmer started his own chiropractic school in Davenport. Later, his son Bartlett Joshua (B.J.) Palmer would take over the school and would oversee the formation of the Palmer College of Chiropractic. B.J. Palmer would go on to perform extensive research in the field of chiropractic and would later author numerous articles and books about the science of chiropractic. He was also the chiropractor who developed many of the spinal analysis and adjusting techniques which are still, for the most part, utilized today.

The Chiropractic Objective

Although all chiropractic practitioners share a common professional title, it should be understood by laypersons that there are two philosophies embedded within this profession. Each philosophy has a unique and special approach when it comes to administering care to patients.

Mixing chiropractic (a slang term used to describe a more allopathic form of chiropractic) has the philosophical objective of treating symptoms of pain along with various conditions. The techniques that are employed by *"chiropractic mixers"* can and do vary greatly. These practitioners will often perform manual manipulations on the spine to improve joint mobility. Manipulations are also commonly performed on other body joints in order to improve mobility and reduce pain. Additional techniques that are used by *"chiropractic mixers"* include, but are not limited to, hot and cold therapies, ultrasound, spinal decompression, acupuncture, nutritional counseling, and cold laser therapy. There are probably additional therapies that I am unintentionally leaving out.

"Mixing chiropractic" mirrors the practice objectives of traditional allopathic medicine with the slight exception that chiropractors do not use drugs or surgery on their patients. *"Chiropractic mixers"* also regularly utilize x-rays, instrumentation, manual palpation and other tools to formulate a proper diagnosis for patients.

Straight chiropractic (traditional chiropractic) is centered on the sole objective of locating and correcting misalignments commonly found in the human spinal column called vertebral subluxations. Traditional chiropractic theory maintains that vertebral segments can and do become misaligned from one another. When such misalignments are present in a person's spine, they can place pressure on corresponding spinal nerves. This condition can impede the function of a given spinal nerve which ultimately causes the human body to operate less efficiently than it would if the nervous system was functioning without any interference. According to traditional chiropractic theory, <u>a person will always function at a much higher level of health</u> when the condition of vertebral subluxation is not present in the spinal column. The absence of subluxation does not guarantee a person good health. There are many factors, besides vertebral subluxation, that determine the overall well being of the human body.

Chiropractic studies have demonstrated that when the nervous system is free of interference, coming from spinal subluxations, the human physiology is more effective in promoting a biological system that can adapt to its ever-changing environment.

Straight (traditional) chiropractors use a variety of methods to analyze the integrity of the spine's alignment including x-rays, instrumentation and hands on palpation of the spinal column. When vertebral subluxations are detected in a patient's spine, through a comprehensive spinal examination, the doctor will make a manual (by hand) adjustment to the spine for the purpose of correcting the misaligned vertebra. Once the spinal subluxation is corrected, the body's nervous system will function more efficiently.

Chiropractors are licensed primary healthcare providers and regardless of a practitioner's philosophical preference, all students are required to take the same number of courses to graduate from an accredited chiropractic college (approximately 5000 hours). All chiropractors must pass the same national board examinations in order to obtain a professional license within the United States.

What's the Best Chiropractic Philosophy?

Over the years, a great number of prospective patients have asked me questions about the professional services I offered. One of the most common questions I have been asked by laypersons considering chiropractic services was, *"What kind of a practitioner should I choose – a mixer or a straight?"* There is not a correct answer to that particular question because each person has different healthcare needs.

Educated healthcare consumers are, without a doubt, going to have a huge advantage over uneducated healthcare consumers when it comes to maintaining their health. Depending on what patients are looking for, from professional chiropractic encounters, the best practitioner might be a mixer, a straight, or both. Only an educated healthcare consumer, that takes the time to do a little research about the practice objectives under examination, will truly know how to select the practitioner that best suits them.

If, as a prospective patient, your goal is to alleviate pain and symptoms, without the use of drugs and invasive surgical procedures, a chiropractic physician *("mixer")* might be the best fit for you. If, on the other hand, you are looking for a way to maintain optimum health, a properly functioning nervous system and the best possible expression of your genetic potential, you should probably consult with a highly qualified straight (traditional) chiropractor.

Some prospective patients consult with both types of doctors. As a prospective patient, you might want to visit a chiropractic physician initially, to resolve an acute condition, and then find a reliable traditional chiropractor that can maintain the integrity of your spine's alignment throughout the entire year.

Understanding Traditional Chiropractic Theory

The human brain sends and receives electrical messages to and from all parts of your body. It is essential that these messages arrive at specific locations, inside of you, throughout your entire life in order for you to remain healthy. These messages travel inside the spinal cord and spinal nerves (Fig1).

The Nervous System

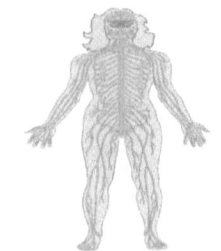

Figure 1 - © OOZ – Fotolia.com

The nervous system is like a giant telephone communication network. It transmits electrical messages that directly affect organs, tissues and cells in the body, and it can also trigger the release of chemical messages that allow other modes of communication to take place within our physiology. Whether it's electrical or chemical communications, the nervous system is behind the transmission of these messages and your body cannot be healthy if the nervous system is not functioning properly.

The spinal cord is very well protected by the spinal bones, and the brain is protected by the skull. Spinal bones (vertebrae) are moveable structures that allow the body flexibility throughout life.

The Spinal Column

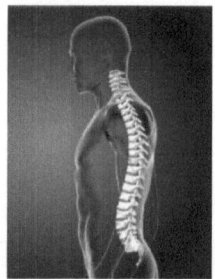

Figure 2 - © JANULLA – Fotolia.com

Because the spinal bones sit on top of one another, they form a long canal of bones where the spinal cord runs through (Fig 2). The spinal nerves that exit from the spinal cord pass between openings that are made on the sides of the spinal bones. Sometimes spinal bones become misaligned from each other and this causes them to place a slight amount of pressure on the spinal nerves. When this happens, the messages that are being transmitted through the nervous system become distorted and this causes problems to occur in the body's physiology.

Traditional chiropractors will nudge the misaligned spinal bones back into their proper anatomical positions by making gentle, manual (by hand) adjustments (Figure 3). This is not done to treat specific conditions of sickness or disease, but rather to correct the misaligned (subluxated) spinal bones. The spinal adjustments help to remove nerve interference and this ultimately allows health to be restored in the body naturally. Many conditions of sickness are then reversed by the body's own inborn recuperative abilities.

A Chiropractic Adjustment

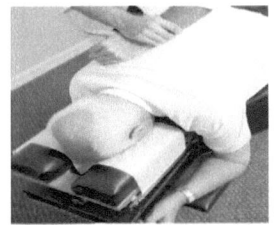

Figure 3 - © Lisa F. Young - Fotolia.com

The Causes of Vertebral Subluxations

The various causes of vertebral subluxations in human beings are too numerous to place on a list. Most subluxations, however, can have their etiology traced back to three distinct categories:

1. Physical Stress
2. Chemical Stress
3. Emotional Stress

Physical stress probably accounts for the formation of most vertebral subluxations found in patients. It is also possible to break down physical stress into *macro* traumas and *micro* traumas.

A *macro* trauma is caused by a major physical event in a person's life such as an automobile accident (Figure 4). This is an injury that has been caused by a major impact, leaving the person in a state of disability with some recovery time to follow. This can certainly have an effect on a person's spinal integrity.

Macro Trauma

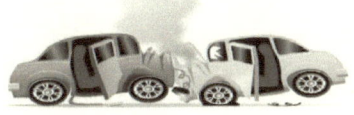

Figure 4 - © abdulsatarid - Fotolia.com

A *micro* trauma is usually caused by repetitive stresses that occur over periods of time. *Micro* traumas often take place in the work place. Occupational stresses that occur repeatedly are often the cause of different micro traumas (Figure 5). Employees of certain jobs might be subjected to work activities which are stressful to them day in and day out for five or six days a week over the course of many years. Speaking on a phone, working on a computer console, lifting heavy materials over and over again can all have a cumulative effect on the status of spinal alignment.

Occupational Stress

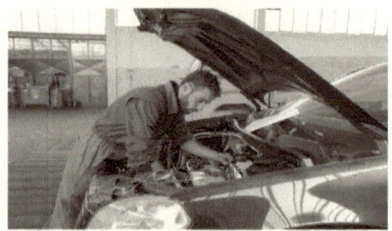

Figure 5 - © olly - Fotolia.com

Recreational activities, such as playing sports or the taking part in hobbies such as wood craft, automotive restoration, and others hobbies, can cause *micro* traumatic insult to the spine.

It is extremely hard to predict when *macro* traumas will occur due to the fact that they are usually received during accidents of some sort. Therefore, the prevention of a *macro* traumatic event is not very likely.

Micro traumas, on the other hand, are very predictable in nature. The problem however, is that people must work to pay bills. It is not practical for patients to quit their jobs in an effort to prevent *micro* traumas from occurring in their lives.

Chemical stress can enter the body and alter biochemistry in the human being. The presence of altered body chemistry can lead to a change in organ and muscle functions. This can then place stress on spinal segments, further compromising the anatomical alignment they share with each other.

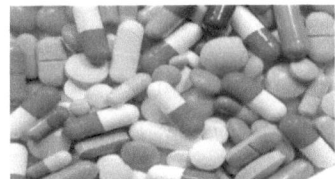

Figure 6 - © Andrzej Tokarski - Fotolia.com

Both prescription and over-the-counter medications can have adverse effects on human physiology as well. Additional chemical stresses can materialize in the forms of various foods which we consume on a regular basis. Preservatives, which are placed in most foods we purchase at the super market, can enter the digestive tract and cause a harmful environment for body physiology. Even foods (organic products) that have not been poisoned with chemical additives can become altered when placed into a microwave oven and nuked for two or three minutes.

The addition of fluoride (a poison) and other toxins that have been added to our drinking water and most brands of tooth paste, marketed within the United States, do not help to reduce people's exposure to chemical stress. Chemicals are everywhere and so therefore it becomes virtually impossible, in today's world, to prevent exposure to this type of stress.

Emotional stress is an additional type of trauma that should not be overlooked as a causal factor for vertebral subluxation formation. The average person is under some type of emotional stress every day of the week. The presence of such emotional tension can cause chemicals to be synthesized in the body which can cause muscle spasms and imbalance. With muscle spasms/imbalance present in the body, an atmosphere is often created that is quite conducive for the genesis of vertebral subluxation.

Unless a person plans to live out the rest of his or her life in a plastic bubble, it would be extremely difficult to prevent repeated exposure to physical, chemical, and emotional stresses. Human beings are constantly challenged by various forms of stress.

It's not stress that actually harms a person. It's an individual's inability to properly adapt to a given form of stress that causes damage to human physiology. Traditional chiropractic theory teaches people that the application of regular chiropractic care enables a human being to be able to adapt to physical, chemical and emotional stresses much more efficiently.

Innate Intelligence

All living things have very unique abilities to be able to adapt to their ever-changing environments. If you think about this for a moment, you will soon realize how amazing life, on our little planet, really is.

Imagine, in your mind's eye, an acorn landing in a field of grass. It becomes naturally embedded in the ground. It receives sunlight and rain and within a short period of time it becomes a tiny sapling. As the years pass, the sapling will grow larger and eventually will mature into a massive, fully grown oak tree that will begin to produce and drop its own acorns. The oak tree is able to survive the toughest elements that are featured in each of the changing seasons. It does all of this, on its own, without a brain. How can this be? The answer is that an acorn and oak tree both contain an inner wisdom, an inborn intelligence which allows it to grow and survive in its immediate environment.

All living things have this inner wisdom that allows life to flourish. In traditional chiropractic, we refer to this inner wisdom as innate intelligence – the inborn wisdom that exists in all living organisms.

As people, we witness examples of innate intelligence on a regular basis. Think about how we eat and digest our food without consciously paying attention to the complex biochemical processes that are involved in accomplishing this task. The human physiology has to break down the food, absorb and assimilate the nutrients, and prepare the leftovers for elimination. We don't have to sit in a room, after eating a large meal, and attempt to figure out the proper amount of chemicals that are necessary to successfully carryout this very important physiological process.

There are also many other examples of innate intelligence that we can observe on a daily basis. The ability of the human eye to adapt and change its point of focus on a given object, in just a few seconds, so that we are able to perceive the surrounding environment in a very clear and unobstructed manner is accomplished through innate intelligence. We don't have to consciously think about calculating the different distances for various objects we encounter so that we can see things properly. The body inherently accomplishes this and other amazing feats, twenty-four hours a day, seven days a week.

The human immune system constantly attempts to keep us healthy by making biochemical adjustments every few seconds as we encounter regularly changing conditions in both our internal and external environments.

A viral or bacterial microbe that has temporarily imposed its will on a living being is no match for the immune system. The inborn intelligence of the body immediately begins to scan the foreign organism for weaknesses and then launches a plan of attack to disable or destroy the offending invader.

In many situations, bacterial and viral microbes are weakened or disabled through heat. The immune system recognizes this weakness and will often create an uncomfortable environment (fever) for these opportunists which aid the body in eliminating infections.

Very often, people make poor healthcare decisions and attempt to interfere with the innate decisions of human physiology. How many individuals do you know that have taken an aspirin, or another drug, in an attempt to lower a fever or to minimize some other annoying symptom? You probably know quite a few folks that have done this – maybe even you!

Just the other day, I was watching a drug commercial about a product that was designed to break up mucus in the airway passages. This drug is an expectorant and it works by thinning out the mucus in the chest and other portions of the body. At first glance, this might seem like a good thing to do. After all, it produces the desired effect (relief) a person suffering with congestion might want. But if we truly understood how smart the human body is, we would rarely interfere with what it is trying to accomplish.

In the case of thinning out mucus in our body, we have to first understand that the inborn intelligence in a human being has a good reason for creating congestion. The body doesn't create thick amounts of copious mucus just for the hell of it. In many situations, the body wants to sequester an active infection from other body areas so that it won't spread and do additional damage. After the immune system successfully destroys the threatening infection, it will reduce the thick mucus in the chest and allow the remnants to be coughed up and expelled. Keep in mind, this is allowed only after the infection has been neutralized.

The problem with taking the expectorant is that the product interferes with the immune system and allows the sequestered infection to be released prematurely through the entire body while it is still active and quite dangerous. This is not a good situation, physiologically speaking, even though it might temporarily give the person some minor relief from the annoying symptoms associated with congestion and an unproductive cough.

Most signs and symptoms, associated with various diseases are nothing more than intelligent attempts by the immune system to rid the body of harmful invaders. Unfortunately, the educated minds of most people in society have been programmed with misinformation when it comes to understanding issues regarding health. A lot of our understanding about health and diseases has come directly from giant petrochemical corporations (drug companies) that have a vested interest in keeping you and I sick throughout our entire lives. The pharmaceutical products that these companies produce do not cure people. Instead, the products block, in a number of ways, the attempts of the immune system to fight off and rid the body of problems that are challenging its overall health.

Millions of Americans are walking around the planet with a condition known as hypertension (elevated blood pressure). If you ask the average person about hypertension, they'll explain to you that high blood pressure is a disease process. They will tell you this because this is what they have been taught by pharmaceutical companies and doctors that have been taught the same nonsense. This misinformation is repeatedly taught at medical schools, which utilize textbooks that have been written by scientists and employees that work for pharmaceutical companies. We are a society filled with repeaters. We keep repeating the same things over and over again without any understanding of what we are repeating!

Hypertension is not a disease! It is a physiological adaptive process which forces blood to reach areas of the body that are not getting adequate blood supplies. The inborn intelligence of the body automatically elevates blood pressure so that people won't die from a stroke or a heart attack. Strokes and heart attacks are caused from an inadequate amount of blood flow to the brain or heart. They are not caused from blood pressure being too high. Very often, strokes and heart attacks will occur in people because the amount of blood going to the heart and brain is insufficient despite the body's attempts to raise blood pressure.

The common protocol to treat patients suffering with hypertension is to place the individuals on medications that will prevent the body's inborn intelligence from raising blood pressure. The drugs actually interfere with the nervous system (they disrupt communication between the brain and other portions of the body) so that the blood pressure cannot be elevated even though it really needs to be raised in order to get a sufficient amount of blood to vital organs and body tissues.

Years ago, a *"normal"* systolic blood pressure reading was widely accepted by the medical community as being 100 + your age. In other words, if you were 75 years old you should have had a systolic blood pressure reading of 175. If you were 40 years old you should have had a systolic blood pressure reading of 140. Systolic blood pressure is a measurement of the blood pressure when the heart is contracting. The other measurement, the bottom number, is known as diastolic blood pressure and is a measurement of the blood pressure when the heart is relaxed. Under the old system, a person that was 80 years old would be considered to have a *"normal"* blood pressure if they produced a reading of 180/80. By today's standards, the same individual would be classified as hypertensive and be prescribed anti-hypertensive medications.

Most medical organizations today are in agreement that a *"normal"* blood pressure reading should be at

115/75. Anything above this level would be classified as hypertension. How convenient this change, in calculating a *"normal"* blood pressure, has been for the pharmaceutical corporations. Their profits originating from selling anti-hypertensive medicines have skyrocketed while people's blood pressures have plummeted along with their health.

In all likelihood, the organizations that conducted the so called *"scientific studies"* that led to the change in how *"normal"* blood pressures are calculated were heavily influenced by the pharmaceutical corporations. By lowering *"normal blood pressure values"* it instantly placed millions of people into a hypertensive category and suggested they be placed on anti-hypertensive medications for the rest of their lives.

The important point that I want my readers to understand is that all living human beings have an inborn (innate) intelligence that constantly strives to keep them alive and well. This intelligence never sleeps, never take a day off from the job and will be with them for as long as they are alive.

Your own innate intelligence always knows what's best for your body, and it is always operating through the very important pathway that keeps you healthy – the human nervous system!

A Typical Chiropractic Visit

The typical office visit to a traditional chiropractor usually takes less than ten minutes out of your busy day. Upon entering the office, a patient is directed to the exam/adjusting room. The patient will be asked to lie down on a slender looking adjusting table. The patient may or may not be gowned, depending on the preference of the practitioner.

The chiropractor will examine and palpate, (lightly touch) with his fingers, the different regions of the patient's spinal column. The spinal column consists of 26 vertebral segments. There are seven cervical vertebrae that make up the area known as the neck; twelve thoracic vertebrae make up the mid back; five lumbar vertebrae create the lower back and there are two bones, the sacrum and coccyx, which form the end of the spinal column. The chiropractor will also examine the two iliac bones, comparing their alignment in relationship to the sacrum, the posterior (back) wall of the pelvis.

Once the chiropractor assesses the alignment of the entire spinal column, he or she will make a chiropractic adjustment (if necessary) to any spinal segments that are subluxated (misaligned from other spinal vertebrae).

Spinal adjustments are usually made by hand or through the use of an adjusting instrument that has a long metal shaft with a small rubber tip on its end. The instrument is usually able to create a quick pulse or thrust of energy that can be directed, very specifically, onto a vertebral segment. The same principle is utilized when a manual (by hand) adjustment is made. During a manual spinal adjustment, the chiropractor will place his hands on a specific vertebral segment and will make a quick thrust into the patient's spine. Once the adjustment is made, and the vertebral segment has been restored to its proper alignment, the chiropractor will palpate the spinal column again to compare the relationship of other vertebrae to one another.

Chiropractic patients are sometimes examined with analytical instruments that will help practitioners to determine if subluxations are present in the spinal column. Most of these tools utilize technologies that can measure heat differentials on both sides of the vertebral column. By comparing temperature readings, in different sections of the spine, chiropractors can calculate what misalignments might be contributing interference to the nervous system.

In certain situations, chiropractors will also utilize spinal radiographs (x-rays) to help assess the alignment of a patient's spine.

During a patient's first visit with a practitioner, a case history is filled out by the patient and reviewed by the chiropractor. A thorough spinal examination is then performed by the chiropractor. After reviewing the results of the examination, the practitioner will decide whether or not to x-ray the patient. Once all exam results have been reviewed, the chiropractor will explain the recommended plan of care that will help the patient achieve the best chiropractic results possible.

Chiropractic, Medicine and the Media

Would you visit a chiropractor if I told you that as a result of getting a chiropractic adjustment you might possibly experience internal bleeding? What about if I told you that you might experience some of the following side effects:

Constipation; decreased sexual desire; diarrhea; dizziness; drowsiness; dry mouth; headaches; increased sweating; lightheadedness when you stand or sit up; liver damage; loss of appetite; nausea; stomach upset; tiredness; trouble sleeping; severe allergic reactions; bloody stools; fainting; fast or irregular heartbeat; hallucinations; memory loss; menstrual period changes; panic attacks, possible development of cancer and or heart disease?

Obviously, you wouldn't want to visit a chiropractor if you knew that these conditions were going to be in your future as a result of getting chiropractic adjustments.

The good news is that chiropractic adjustments don't cause any of the previously mentioned effects/conditions. The side effects I have listed are caused by commonly purchased over-the-counter and prescription drugs.

The same people that wouldn't visit a chiropractor to avoid these side effects will continue to purchase and take very dangerous drugs.

WHY?

It is widely believed by many healthcare practitioners that chiropractic adjustments improve the function of your nervous system and promote a better functioning immune system that ultimately allows people to be a lot healthier than they would be without chiropractic care. In spite of this good news, most people avoid getting under chiropractic care. It's a fact! Most people do not use the services of a chiropractor because they have been incorrectly informed (by pharmaceutical corporations and the news companies that promote their toxic products) that chiropractic is dangerous or not based on *"real science."* Even worse, many people have been programmed by the media to believe that chiropractic is only a limited therapy for neck and back pain.

For a number of years I taught a course at a chiropractic college that dealt with the subject of communications. One of the many things I discussed in that forum was the incredible power the media holds over the general population. It amazed the students in my class how easily people were influenced by various media products.

Another interesting caveat we thoroughly covered was the topic of media ownership and the uncomfortable fact that a few very large corporations owned the entire media playground. At that particular time (2006), only five companies maintained a virtual monopoly on the production and distribution of every piece of news that was being reported. It was quite apparent to me and my students that some very wealthy elitists, and the corporations they owned, were using the media to paint a false perception of reality for the rest of the world.

The large corporations, through the media assets they have acquired, are effectively controlling the perceptions of many human beings (Figure 7). The poisoning of the human mind, through media programming, has been taking place for a very long time.

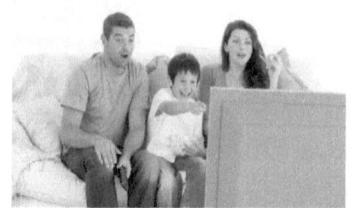

Figure 7 - © WavebreakMediaMicro - Fotolia.com

The local and national media are routinely used to influence and control the way people in society think about many things including healthcare, chiropractic and the practice of traditional medicine. Allopathy is regularly described by the mainstream media as a panacea for all illness. Chiropractic, on the other hand, is regularly described by the media as a controversial form of alternative healthcare that borders on being credible and unscientific.

Every single day, on virtually any news broadcast, there is a time slot dedicated to the next miracle drug or breakthrough to manage cancer or some other plague overtaking humanity.

The various presentations that showcase the medical profession, through media products and associated props, as ultra scientific are very clever. The customary *"white lab coat"* is usually worn by doctors and researchers being interviewed on television. The image of a *"white lab coat"* has been painstakingly etched into our minds. It yells out to all of us and says, *"The individual wearing the white garment is honest and he or she is a scientist!"* People actually feel more comfortable when they see a lab technician or a doctor wearing something white while looking into a microscope. Other props, like a stethoscope or reflex hammer, are also worn by medical doctors when being interviewed on national television programs because these tools are easily recognized by the viewing audience and, on a subconscious level, speak to members of society telling them, *this person should be respected and knows what he or she is speaking about.* It all leads back to cultivating and finely shaping a person's perception of reality. Media products accomplish this important objective for the pharmaceutical corporations.

"Trust Me… I'm A Doctor!"

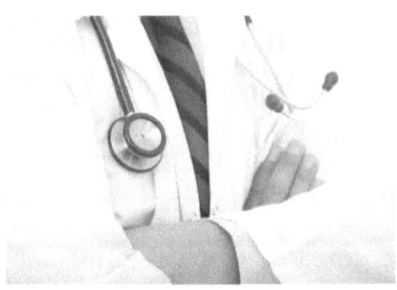

Figure 8 - © khz - Fotolia.com

Over the years, the medical wardrobe and its associated props have been carefully carved into the psyche of the American public, in an effort to garner society's unwarranted respect for the Medical Establishment. Television news programs, sitcoms, movies, magazine articles and other media products have methodically unleashed an amazing brainwashing campaign on an unsuspecting viewing audience.

Foundations and organizations, ad nauseam, have been developed by the Medical Establishment (secretly funded by the pharmaceutical corporations) in an effort to regularly promote awareness about various diseases to the public. Walkathons; races for a cure; parades and professional sports leagues that outfit their players in specially colored uniforms, during a certain month to promote an awareness about a specific disease, are just a few of the ways people have been hoodwinked into believing that traditional allopathic protocols have been implemented into society by the Medical Establishment for no reason other than to help patients.

In reality, the foundations and organizations that have been created to promote awareness about specific diseases are doing a great job in making sure the lucrative disease industry never disappears.

I know that this is a hard pill to swallow for many people because the conclusion one comes to, from reading this information, is very disturbing. The mere mentioning of this type of material also speaks volumes about how absolutely awful certain corporations really are. It is uncomfortable for many people to think that others would have no problem profiting from the misery of others. But this is exactly what is happening in the healthcare environment. The pharmaceutical industry has only one concern – profit! They do not care about the health and well being of healthcare consumers.

If you examine the various foundations that have the names of the diseases they are supporting/promoting built within their organization's title, you will see that these entities are financed and promoted, at all of their official events, websites, etc., by pharmaceutical companies that specialize in offering the drugs that are currently used to manage the different maladies in question. You'll also notice that the pharmaceutical companies never promise a cure, just long term management of each disease process. This is an absolutely ingenious plan that was implemented long ago by the pharmaceutical corporations. They have given birth to foundations (support groups) that engage in regular annual campaigns, which have the sole objective of promoting awareness to compromised healthcare consumers about poisonous drugs that are available to manage a specific ailment.

Many of the disease processes currently plaguing humanity could have easily been eradicated by natural methods, but the pharmaceutical companies will never allow this to happen.

Many of the food products we regularly consume today are being produced or prepared by companies that are owned and operated by larger companies that have direct ties to the pharmaceutical corporations. It's pretty apparent that the larger parent corporations don't want to get rid of the diseases they are already profiting from. Is it possible that they want to create more diseases? Is it also possible that these corporations are responsible for the current plagues already terrorizing humanity?

In my considered opinion, I think there's a good possibility that a lot of these diseases have been designed and purposely unleashed on society so that companies can earn profits. Many of the giant corporations in question are directly or indirectly responsible for genetically modifying our foods. When you visit the supermarket, it's almost impossible to find products that have not been laced with artificial sweeteners and other harmful ingredients.

Scientists believe that many of these substances are toxic and making people very ill.

Anytime a person has the courage to research an alternative approach to health through the vehicles of nutrition, naturopathy, homeopathy, chiropractic, etc., they are instantly greeted with warnings from websites and media spokespersons posing disingenuously as members of consumer watch groups.

I want my readers to understand that healthcare is big business and it generates billions of dollars in profits on an annual basis. If you were only permitted to learn one essential item about running a successful business, you would want to know that it is the goal of every company to constantly increase its profits while trying to find new and creative ways to expand existing business. In a nutshell, you want more customers who need or utilize your products and services.

We Make Money and Cure Absolutely Nothing!

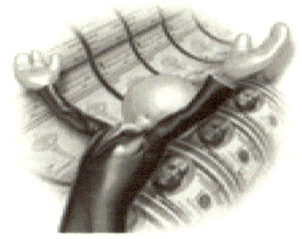

Figure 9 - © Scott Maxwell - Fotolia.com

49

Most people believe the healthcare industry (pharmaceutical industry) is in the business of getting sick people well. It is this be**lie**f that allows the overall health of our population to continuously decline a little more each year.

As the years pass, it seems as though more terrifying diseases are arriving on the scene. *Autoimmune disorders, Cancer, AIDS, Diabetes, cardiovascular problems, viruses*, and many other serious health conditions continue to make their way into our lives. On the surface, it is made to look like the pharmaceutical companies are burning the oil day and night in an attempt to find a cure for these deadly diseases. Can you picture all the scientists in a very sophisticated laboratory setting, donned in white gowns, peering down into rows of microscopes? It's the hope of the average person that one of these scientists will produce a cure for *Cancer* or for one of the other previously mentioned plagues. Don't hold your breath! It's not going to happen in your lifetime or in your children's lifetime!

Do you know how much money is made by pharmaceutical companies each year for the treatment of *cancer*? What about for the treatment of *AIDS, diabetes, heart disease, hypertension, influenza, the common cold, headaches, depression, or rheumatoid arthritis?* The answer is billions of dollars. That's right – billions of dollars are earned every year by pharmaceutical companies that have patents on various drugs that are used to treat symptoms associated with these deadly diseases.

Pharmaceutical companies depend on these diseases to make large profits. It wouldn't be very smart for a pharmaceutical company to conduct research that would lead to a cure for a specific disease. Why would a company want to destroy a cash cow?

Instead, these giant companies use other assets they have procured, such as international media companies, and they spend large sums of money launching campaigns designed to make you and I believe that real science is quackery and quackery is real science. This is classic "*Alice in Wonderland*" trickery and you are presently in kindergarten and just beginning to discover how deep the rabbit hole actually goes.

Let's "Google" Chiropractic

Several years ago I was surfing the Internet and decided to "Google" the word chiropractic. On the very top of the search page was a link to a website that claimed to be owned and operated by a consumer watch group. This website, at first glance, appeared to be dedicated to warning healthcare consumers about unscrupulous alternative healthcare practitioners. Upon further and more detailed inspection, I discovered that the website was actually designed to discredit any holistic healthcare discipline that veered away from traditional, allopathic rationale. This discrediting theme was focused on the practices of nutritional therapy, naturopathy, homeopathy, acupuncture, chiropractic, and some alternative healthcare modalities.

Realizing the extensive damage a webpage of this nature could do to the chiropractic profession, I attempted to leave commentary for the site's administrator asking that the material be removed from the Internet. As I had expected, there was never a reply from the site administrator and the web content has remained active on the Internet to this day.

The author(s) of this website claim that their mission statement is to identify healthcare professionals that are dangerous and pose a threat to the public. I guess that I should be grateful for their service, but I am not. I am saddened because I believe that the website in question is most likely financed by multinational pharmaceutical corporations and the people that write for this forum, and others like it, are nothing more than paid shills for them.

According to the author(s) of the website and related web pages that can be traced back to the mother site, anything that promotes chiropractic wellness care; subluxation correction; chiropractic care for children; negative views against traditional medicine; anti-vaccination ideas, anti-fluoridation ideas, non-traditional approaches to fighting cancer or any other serious diseases should be immediately dismissed as unscientific and considered a threat to the general public. After reading the content on this website, I thought I was going to throw up.

As members of society, we are regularly encouraged by the Medical Establishment to behave like good little children, not to make waves and obey the advice of conventional medicine. Those brave souls that venture "outside the box" of conventional thinking, more often than not, will face a heavy dose of criticism from an unforgiving society which never considers questioning the Medical Establishment or leaving the confinement of such a well defined and protected safe zone.

Time and time again I have listened to anti-chiropractic spokespeople state their pathetic cases that chiropractic and the vertebral subluxation theory are not scientifically provable. The weak arguments that are presented by the skeptics are largely based on illogical thoughts about vertebral subluxations not being able to be viewed on x-rays (radiographs).

In reality, their arguments are not accurate. Vertebral subluxation degeneration is very visible on radiographs. Degenerative Joint Disease (DJD) in the spinal column, otherwise known as osteoarthritis of the spine, is caused exclusively from spinal misalignments. Although the actual nerve compression component that takes place when a vertebral subluxation is present might not be observable when viewing plain radiographs, the damaging effects caused from the structural misalignments are quite obvious to even the most untrained eye.

As a former faculty member at a chiropractic college, I had direct access to research materials and regularly conversed with colleagues that performed chiropractic research. I have viewed, during my career, numerous medical and chiropractic journals that have published studies demonstrating the validity of vertebral subluxations. There is no doubt that research studies have been performed and confirm vertebral subluxations can and do occur in the human spinal column.

The reason these studies are never published in the most prestigious medical journals in the world is because they have been purposely excluded by pharmaceutical companies. Any form of research that promotes the concepts or ideas that health can be achieved without pharmaceutical products seems to be immediately discarded or hidden. In addition, any study that does not promote the use of drugs or traditional pharmaceutical protocols, when discussing health, is also usually dismissed as unscientific. Chiropractic, the largest, drugless, primary healthcare profession in the world, falls into this category and is therefore aggressively attacked by the large pharmaceutical corporations and every resource they have at their disposal. One of those resources would be websites designed to look like they represent legitimate consumer watch groups, supposedly looking out for our best interests. Don't you feel protected?

Please Don't Mention the Vaccines!

If you want to infuriate the traditional medical establishment, just start talking negatively about the sacred subject of medical vaccinations.

Officially, the chiropractic profession does not have an opinion about medical vaccinations. The vaccination topic is a medical issue that falls outside the practice scope of the chiropractor. Nevertheless, many chiropractors have strong opinions about this subject and they have voiced those opinions in public forums. Because many chiropractors tend to be outspoken and unafraid of voicing their opinions about this controversial subject, it seems that the entire chiropractic profession has been targeted for elimination by the traditional Medical Establishment.

I have always believed that if chiropractors had been less vocal through the years about the dangers of vaccines, the medical profession would have been a lot less motivated to destroy our profession. The rationale for this statement is centered on my strong opinion that the vaccination campaign, more than anything else in traditional allopathy, is the *"Holy Grail"* of medicine.

A lot of very smart people have extensively researched the vaccination topic. There are loads of articles and books that have been authored by medical doctors, physiologists and other scientists with impressive credentials. Some of their writings have warned the public to steer clear from vaccines. At the very end of this book, I have listed some publications and websites so that readers can access additional information about this important subject.

Take This Poison… It's Good For You!

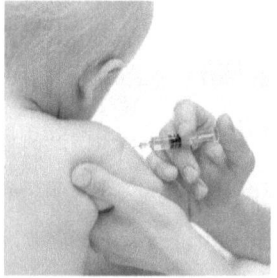

Figure 10 - © Dmitry Naumov - Fotolia.com

At the very center of the vaccination controversy is the recent anger of many families that believe there's a connection between vaccines and autism. People have been asking for compensation for damages stemming from immunization injuries to their children for many years. This is not a new concept by any stretch of the imagination.

Pharmaceutical companies have had to pay out compensation in the past in an effort to settle suits generated from vaccination injuries to small children. It appears, when one reviews the large number of claims being made today, that a lot of children might be getting needlessly harmed from vaccines. This is not something that can be hidden any longer as the complaints have been recently showcased on the mainstream news networks and the accusatory finger has been pointed in the face of the Medical Establishment for their involvement in causing more harm than good when it comes to the vaccine issue.

Please keep in mind that it is every person's responsibility to be knowledgeable about healthcare issues. Many people in the healthcare arena believe that vaccinations are responsible for quite a few of the healthcare problems that have recently surfaced in modern society. I wholeheartedly agree with them. Nevertheless, you should remember to make healthcare decisions for you and your family members only after carefully studying available literature about a specific topic and then consulting with various members of the healthcare community.

I tell patients that I take care of in my private practice where to search for information about this controversial subject. I have personally read many books, articles, and journals about vaccinations and I try to pass on the information, which I have uncovered throughout the years, to my patients. When you give people the proper resources to make intelligent decisions about their own healthcare needs, you are fulfilling your role as a doctor. You are also helping to teach your patients that health originates from within the body and that the acquisition of healthcare knowledge, through the reading of books, is an essential component in keeping the members of our society at an optimal level of health.

Now that I have written the standard disclaimer, explaining that readers should make an informed choice about taking vaccines by reading as much information as possible, let me tell you my personal opinion about what I think is taking place. I think vaccines are harming people. I believe these very dangerous drugs are making people weaker, sicker, and vulnerable to diseases they would otherwise not have to contend with. I also believe these medicines do not create immunity and that the vaccine ingredients are toxic beyond belief and bad for all human beings.

Much of the literature I've read, during my career as a healthcare practitioner, leads me to believe that vaccinations are probably responsible for the large number of people suffering with autoimmune disorders. In my opinion, these diseases are more prevalent in society than ever before. Autoimmune diseases require long term medical management through the use of extremely expensive and dangerous drugs. The drugs that are often used to treat many of these conditions suppress the human immune system and almost guarantee the patients taking the products a future littered with severe medical complications down the road. This is a very profitable situation for pharmaceutical companies. This, in my opinion, is why the Medical Establishment has pushed vaccinations so aggressively on all members of society.

In summary, I believe vaccines actually weaken the human immune system and set up the compromised individual for a lifelong dependency on drugs. I don't believe vaccines prevent diseases. In my opinion, vaccines prevent the natural expression of health and ensure the Medical Establishment a never ending supply of customers that will require toxic drugs for the rest of their lives.

It never made much sense to me why human beings would need synthetic poisons injected into their bodies in order to protect themselves from diseases. The entire concept always seemed odd even before I studied microbiology and had an extensive healthcare education.

Because chiropractors and other alternative healthcare providers have warned the public about these dangerous drugs, they have been singled out by the Medical Establishment and have been made to look like quacks. The best way to minimize damage coming from another healthcare profession that's pointing out obvious flaws in your own profession is to discredit the people or profession that is creating the problem. This might be a daunting task unless you had access to unlimited resources. If you owned or had tremendous influence over media corporations, insurance companies, accrediting agencies involved in approving and regulating curricula for chiropractic colleges, as well as many other assets that are too numerous to list; the dirty deed could possibly be pulled off.

The giant pharmaceutical corporations that are a big part of the Medical Establishment, in my opinion, have those unlimited resources and they have become so powerful that it is virtually impossible to stop the abuse that is currently taking place.

My friends and colleagues have asked me why I continue to write about corruption and conspiracies that are too big to stop and too embedded within our culture to question. My answer to them is that I have to try and educate others about what I know to be the truth.

The Benefits of Traditional Medicine

In this book, I have been very critical of the medical establishment and the pharmaceutical corporations that I believe have hijacked the medical industry. I want readers to understand that my criticism of the Medical Establishment does not mean that I believe modern medicine has no importance in our everyday lives. Quite the contrary, I believe the medical profession has an important role in modern society.

If I was seriously injured in an auto accident, I'd want to be taken to an emergency trauma center and placed under the close supervision of highly skilled medical personnel.

If I ever needed to have an organ patched, some arteries fixed, or my finger reattached to my hand, I'd want to be in the company of qualified surgeons that would be able to get the job done and save my life.

Sometimes, the human body becomes extremely compromised from various forms of stress, and we need to take drugs. Pain killers, antibiotics, and other pharmaceutical products can, in certain situations, be beneficial to human beings if they are carefully prescribed by medical doctors for limited periods of time. I recognize this fact and wanted my readers to understand where I am coming from in regards to a healthcare perspective. I am not anti-medical!

The fact that the profession of medicine is an important component of society should not diminish the importance of teaching people some of the serious problems associated with our current healthcare system. Although allopathy can produce some definite health benefits for certain patients, there is also the potential for it to harm patients receiving treatment for long term chronic disorders.

I believe that traditional medical care can be beneficial if it is used in a limited manner, to stabilize patients that have suffered traumas or require surgical procedures after less invasive and natural types of care have been completely exhausted. Practiced in this way, modern medicine can play an important role in helping people regain their level of health and well being.

Debunking the Debunkers

Throughout the Medical Establishment's long history of trying to damage the credibility of the chiropractic profession, debunking agents or so called *"experts"* have been hired by the *"powers that be"* to make chiropractic and its practitioners appear to look like quacks. The agents have given interviews, written books, constructed websites, and participated in other campaigns that directly reached healthcare consumers and helped to create false perceptions for people about chiropractic.

The funding of these campaigns has come from giant pharmaceutical corporations. It is very difficult to point fingers and name names because paid shills are not going to admit to the fact that they're on the payroll of a specific company, working to undermine or destroy chiropractic. It's important to understand that chiropractic is not the only alternative healthcare profession that has been attacked. Anything that has gone against the grain of conventional medical theory has been fair game!

Debunking agents are presently used everyday and in many different ways. Pretty much anything that challenges the accepted norms of what society perceives as being reality would be applicable. For example, if a large minority of the population began to suddenly question the authenticity of something that was being reported by the government or the mainstream media, debunking agents, employed by the *powers that be*, are always ready to spring into action. These people, through the implementation of strategic campaigns, can absolutely minimize the damage being caused by a controversial voice within the population base. The agents can make sure that the majority of the population continues to perceive reality the way that the government or media originally intended. For the purpose of this book, I'll only discuss this topic as it pertains to healthcare and more specifically, chiropractic.

Giant pharmaceutical companies have a lot at stake in this very lucrative game. In order for these companies to remain profitable and powerful in the future, society must continue to believe in certain erroneous concepts like vaccines keep people healthy. Pharmaceutical companies have many assets to ensure that their paradigm; the only way to maintain health is through suppressive drug therapies, is always protected and stays in play.

Alternative healthcare has always been a threat to the Medical Establishment. Because of this, it has been an important goal of traditional medicine to employ scientists and other professionals that could appear credible when attempting to write or convey damaging remarks about a particular modality or profession within the framework of alternative healthcare.

As I wrote earlier, quite a few websites have been designed to make potential viewers wary of chiropractic, as well as other alternative healthcare services. It becomes easy to spot the disingenuous web addresses once you know what you're looking for. The paid shills writing for *"Big Pharma,"* usually copy and repeat the same misinformation on different web locations.

The oldest trick in the book (and all the chiropractic debunkers use this tactic) is to claim traditional chiropractic (vertebral subluxation correction) has not undergone scientific, double blind studies and is therefore not a valid form of healthcare.

To begin to understand how totally flawed double-blind studies are when applied to the traditional chiropractic model, you have to first understand what these tests are actually trying to accomplish. Double blind studies have been designed to test the effectiveness of different drugs on patients. What the double blind studies are really testing is the effectiveness of a drug's ability to cover up or block symptoms in the human body.

As I have already explained, earlier in this book, symptoms are not caused by the disease process but rather by the body's immune system, in an attempt to disable the disease process. An example of this is a common fever. The fever that takes place during a bacterial or viral infection is attempting to destroy the microbe making the person ill. The double-blind study is actually measuring how effective a certain drug is in preventing the body from working as it should. If we used, for example, the fever scenario in a double-blind study, we would have to administer samples of medications to several patients that had fevers. Both the patients and the persons administering the drugs would be blind to which samples were the fever reducing drugs and which samples were sugar pills or placebos. The study would examine how effective certain samples were in reducing fever—the desired effect coming from the drug.

While double blind studies might be a useful tool when it comes to measuring how well drugs are harming the overall health of an individual, they are a totally unreliable ruler when used to measure the effectiveness of a chiropractic adjustment being administered to a patient for the purpose of correcting a vertebral subluxation.

Traditional chiropractic has nothing to do with addressing or blocking symptoms. Traditional chiropractic seeks to eliminate the cause of a serious problem by removing a major interference from the nervous system. This translates into a very beneficial result for the person involved however, the results would be impossible to measure through a double blind study. The double-blind study could never be applied to the traditional chiropractic model because these studies are only valuable when measuring changes in symptoms. Unfortunately, that's what most of traditional medicine is all about. It has the objective of covering up certain physiological expressions associated with health conditions and never addresses the causes of these problems.

By virtue of the double-blind study, science has already proven that medicine, and the drugs it utilizes, are most effective in blocking the body's natural abilities to fight off diseases. This is why traditional medicine has never cured one single disease.

Once you eliminate the double blind study argument, the skeptics/shills writing the propaganda on various websites begin to point out that chiropractic should be classified as a pseudoscience because the profession's practitioners have dangerous ideas about conventional medical theories. On this point I would definitely agree with the debunkers. Many chiropractic practitioners have routinely pointed out a lot of gaping holes in the Medical Establishment's protocols for the management of various diseases. This is a dangerous scenario for the medical profession.

Some dangerous chiropractic ideas, according to the debunkers, that I can think of right off the top of my head are anti-vaccination and anti-fluoridation campaigns. Chiropractors have had a lot to say about the dangers associated with vaccines and water fluoridation. Both of these practices are very controversial and can, in the opinions of many healthcare professionals worldwide, cause irreparable damage to the human immune system.

My advice to prospective patients that stumble upon anti-chiropractic websites, and other related literature, is to realize that this type of content is being purposely placed in the public domain by the Medical Establishment to make healthcare consumers believe that chiropractic and many forms of alternative healthcare are based on pseudoscientific principles.

Chiropractic is a fully licensed form of healthcare in all fifty states. Government agencies wouldn't license healthcare professionals if their professional objectives were based on unscientific principles!

Are Chiropractic Adjustments Safe?

If you listen to some of the propaganda that is delivered through the mainstream media, you might develop the general perception that chiropractic is a dangerous profession. You need to keep remembering that media campaigns are designed to fool laypersons so that they do not buy into alternative healthcare philosophies. Everything must be authenticated by the mainstream gatekeepers for it to be considered valid and safe for public consumption.

Once again, the reality of the situation is often different than what most people perceive the situation to be. According to insurance actuaries *(people who calculate the level of risk in an insurance policy)*, the practice of traditional chiropractic is one of the safest healthcare professions in the world. Many doctors of chiropractic pay only a few hundred dollars a year to secure their professional liability policies. On the other side of the coin, many medical healthcare practitioners pay hundreds of thousands of dollars during the course of a single year just so they can have liability coverage.

As I indicated in an earlier chapter, many medically backed agencies have disingenuously posed as consumer watch groups. These agencies have repeatedly painted the chiropractic adjustment as a dangerous procedure. Considering that within the last fifty years only a minimal number of patient injuries have been attributed to chiropractic procedures and that insurance premiums for chiropractic liability policies are the lowest of any primary healthcare providers, it is almost laughable that organized medicine is able to continuously suggest that chiropractic is a direct threat to the safety of the American healthcare consumer.

In August of 1987, the American Medical Association, the American College of Radiologists, and the American College of Surgeons were all found guilty of conspiring to eliminate the profession of chiropractic by Federal Judge Susan Getzendanner of the United States District court. *(Wilk et al v. AMA et al, No. 90-542 a record of public information)* Because traditional medicine, with the help of other organizations, attempted to destroy another competitive healthcare profession, a high level of skepticism should be used by laypersons when reading anti-chiropractic literature originating from traditional medical sources.

Strangely enough, most people were never made aware of the fact that there was a conspiracy against chiropractic and that organized medicine was responsible for designing the entire plot. It is the common belief of many chiropractors that very heavily funded anti-chiropractic campaigns are still being launched today, behind the scenes, by organized medicine.

The chiropractic adjustment is probably one of the best kept secrets within the entire healthcare industry. If traditional medicine and the pharmaceutical industry continue to have their way, the chiropractic adjustment will most likely remain a secret indefinitely.

Do Chiropractic Adjustments Hurt?

One of the biggest fears people have about chiropractic is that the spinal adjustments are painful. There are many misconceptions by laypersons about this subject as well as how chiropractors perform these adjustments on their patients.

The spinal adjustment is a very precise technical procedure that is accomplished manually or with the use of an adjusting instrument. Adjustments are very specific as they are capable of moving one vertebral segment that is subluxated back into its proper anatomical alignment while leaving other bones, which are not subluxated, untouched.

Adjustments, for the most part, are painless and many chiropractic patients report to chiropractors, family members, and friends that the procedures actually feel good. Only a minimal amount of force is administered into a patient's spine by the doctor when making a spinal correction.

Doctors of chiropractic spend thousands of hours studying a variety of techniques that have been designed to help the chiropractor complete his or her professional objective of locating, analyzing and correcting vertebral subluxations.

The actual chiropractic adjusting techniques often look relatively easy to perform to the untrained layperson. This is another false perception about chiropractic that the lay community has developed throughout the years. There are some very important technical skills that a chiropractic student must master in order to become proficient in delivering various adjusting techniques. Obviously, a doctor's knowledge of physics and spinal bio-dynamics are the major determining factors in how successful a specific technique package will be performed or delivered in the actual practice setting.

Doctors of chiropractic will often spend many additional hours attending technique seminars after graduating from college in order that they can continue to perfect their adjusting skills. The chiropractic adjustment is placed on the tallest of pedestals by chiropractors. There are probably very few practitioners, within any organized profession, that devote as much time as chiropractors do in developing an individual component within their chosen trade.

In summary, chiropractic adjustments are very technical procedures that require a great deal of skill to perform properly. When utilized by a truly competent chiropractor, they are both safe and painless for patients.

Chiropractic versus Medicine

Traditional chiropractic and medicine have different professional objectives. The profession of chiropractic has the ultimate goal of maintaining a person's health by removing a type of interference to the nervous system which inhibits the true expression of health in all human beings.

The profession of medicine attempts to cure various diseases that are affecting the body by prescribing certain medications that reverse or oppose physiological processes occurring in the body and also through the application of surgical procedures which attempt to remove or repair compromised human tissues.

Traditional chiropractic has a vitalistic philosophy which adheres to the premise that health comes from within the body or from the inside out. This philosophy acknowledges the fact that all human beings have inherent abilities to maintain their own healthy existence and that a disruption of health is caused internally. Traditional chiropractic states that if health is lost from within the body it must logically be restored from the inside out.

Medicine has a different philosophy and it claims that the human body is weak and must constantly have its health maintained from the outside in. According to modern medicine, a human being must have an assortment of vaccines and other preventive medicinal compounds in order to build up the immune system.

In summary, traditional chiropractic works with the controlling laws of nature and physiology while organized medicine (allopathy) attempts to go against the controlling laws of nature and physiology.

What About the Children?

One of the most frequently asked questions by laypersons is whether or not they should bring their children to the chiropractor for care. Infants and young children should definitely be under the care of a qualified chiropractor. Some of the first subluxations that show up in the spine appear very early in a child's life.

One of the most damaging forces children will ever face occurs during the actual process that brings them into this world – childbirth. Not so much the process that was designed and activated by nature, but rather the procedure designed by organized medicine and man's educated mind. A procedure that places great stress on the cervical spine of the newborn and sets the stage for an abundance of health disorders over the entire lifetime of the individual.

The birthing process is very traumatic for the mother and the child. In the case of the child, the twisting and pulling on the head and cervical spine creates a very good chance for spinal subluxations to occur.

In general, children are much more active than adults and they are constantly being exposed to many physical stresses that originate from the everyday things that kids take part in.

A child's immune system is regularly being fine tuned to its immediate environment. In addition, biology and science have demonstrated through research that the nervous system plays an integral role in how well the immune system within a developing child is functioning. Chiropractic care is going to help children maintain the integrity of their spinal alignment and this is reason enough to bring a child to the chiropractor. Proper spinal alignment will also help the nervous system to work without interference coming from spinal subluxations and so it becomes quite easy to understand why parents should regularly bring their children to the chiropractor's office.

Am I Subluxated?

A lot of chiropractic patients incorrectly believe they can tell when they are subluxated. Most of the spinal nerves that pass through the vertebrae, on their way to various parts of the body, are not responsible for delivering pain sensations to the brain. In other words, people are unable to sense when there is pressure being exerted on many of the spinal nerves.

I have been a practicing chiropractor for many years and I am unable to determine when my own body is subluxated and in need of a chiropractic adjustment. The only sure way for people to know if they are subluxated would be to visit a chiropractor and undergo a proper chiropractic spinal examination. Unfortunately, vertebral subluxations are usually painless. Through the years, this condition has been nicknamed *"the silent killer"* because of how it lurks in a person's spine robbing them each day of their true genetic potential to be healthy.

Traditional chiropractors continue to take part in local and national campaigns that have the common objective of educating laypersons living within communities around the country to regularly utilize chiropractic services. If these campaigns are successful, there will be less people in society that will be subluxated and a really serious condition, which adversely affects the human nervous system, will finally be addressed.

What About Back Pain?

Back pain and many other symptomatic conditions that can make the life of a patient less comfortable are not the professional focal points for traditional chiropractors. Traditional chiropractic has only one objective which is to locate, analyze and correct vertebral subluxations in a person's spinal column. The rationale for doing this is simply explained by reiterating the fact that a subluxation can create a type of interference within a person's nervous system which can impede that individual's overall level of health.

Regardless of whether or not patients have specific conditions challenging them, they are always better off without the presence of vertebral subluxations in their spines. Subluxations are capable of inhibiting the full expression of health in any individual. Many traditional healthcare objectives focus exclusively on treating specific conditions/symptoms that afflict members of society. Traditional chiropractic recognizes the inherent recuperative abilities of living beings and works in harmony with those healing capabilities.

It is easy for some chiropractic practitioners to lose focus of the bigger picture within healthcare by focusing exclusively on patients' symptomatic complaints. While it is true that patients occasionally report to their doctors that symptoms are alleviated after starting a program of chiropractic care, it is vitally important laypersons understand that conditions of sickness and disease have many causes that are not directly attributable to vertebral subluxations.

Traditional chiropractic does not attempt to deliver individual cures for specific ailments but instead looks to remove a type of interference from the nervous system which inhibits the body's inborn ability to maintain its own health naturally.

The problem with thinking of chiropractic care as a *"mechanical aspirin"* is that many spinal subluxations do not produce pain or other noticeable symptoms. There are many instances where patients are subluxated and not aware of what is taking place inside their bodies.

In my professional opinion, there has never been a situation where a person directly benefited from the presence of vertebral subluxations in his or her spinal column. The vertebral subluxation, always and without exception, presents a challenge for the human body to be able to adapt to its ever changing environment.

Keep in mind that traditional chiropractic can help correct spinal subluxations when detected in a particular patient. On the other hand, the presence or absence of a patient's back pain is considered irrelevant by the focused, traditional chiropractor.

Why are there so Many Techniques?

There are quite a few different techniques used within the chiropractic profession. Many laypersons often incorrectly assume that there are different techniques designed to address specific conditions. For example, I have been asked over the years by certain patients to administer the same adjustment that I had performed on them at a previous visit. These patients believed that a specific technique was responsible for removing their indigestion, sinusitis or other equally annoying conditions.

It's important that patients and laypersons understand that techniques are simply the tools that a chiropractor uses to correct subluxations within their spines. The subluxation is what a chiropractor must focus on finding. Through the application of a carefully selected technique package; the practitioner is able to aid the body in correcting a potentially devastating condition that robs the human physiology of its natural ability to be healthy.

Some patients present unique anatomical challenges for practitioners. In certain situations, a patient might not be able to turn his head in a certain direction or he might be unable to assume a certain position on the adjusting table. It is therefore necessary for chiropractors to know a wide variety of techniques in order to be able to accommodate the patients that enter the office setting.

Keep in mind that there is not a special technique that chiropractors use to treat certain conditions in the body. There are however, a rather large number of dependable techniques that are very successful in correcting the one and only problem that traditional chiropractors address – the vertebral subluxation.

Can Chiropractic Cause Arthritis?

Arthritis is a general term that describes a disease process that often occurs in human beings and other animals. This disease can affect the joints in the body and is characterized by various degrees of inflammation. Most forms of arthritis are caused by misalignments of bony joints within the skeletal system or from a systemic disorder (rheumatoid arthritis) that affects the clear synovial fluid which normally helps to lubricate and nourish the body's bony joints. People with rheumatoid arthritis have synovial fluid that irritates and attacks the bony joints within the body.

Systemic forms of arthritis (rheumatoid arthritis) are thought to originate from an immune system that is not working properly. Autoimmune disorders cause the body's immune system to work in a non productive manner. The joints in the body often become inflamed and eventually, after a number of years, begin to exhibit a number of degenerative changes.

The most common form of arthritis is known as osteoarthritis, which is caused from misaligned bony joints. Very often, misalignments within the bony joints of the body are caused from physical traumas. Once the bones become misaligned, the body makes an attempt to realign them by causing muscles that are attached to the bones to contract. In many instances, the intelligence of the body is successful in correcting the misalignments. In the event the body is unable to resolve the misalignments, through the contraction of muscles, the intelligence of the body will initiate another process which will attempt to cement the bones, in a fixed position, preventing any further problems in the future.

The objective of traditional chiropractic is to maintain the integrity of the spine's alignment which promotes a healthy nervous system. Since the nervous system directly affects a person's immune system, it would be logical to assume that the correction of vertebral subluxations would have a positive effect on people having immune system disorders. It is therefore not logical to assume that chiropractic care would be responsible for causing rheumatoid arthritis.

Osteoarthritis is directly caused from bony misalignments and a vertebral subluxation is definitely a type of joint misalignment that occurs within the spinal column. Chiropractors correct spinal misalignments (vertebral subluxations) and therefore reduce the likelihood of any arthritic degeneration in the spine. Regular chiropractic care would therefore greatly reduce the chances of arthritis showing up in a person's spine. The misconception that chiropractic care can cause arthritis is both illogical and physiologically impossible.

Is Chiropractic Addictive?

Laypersons commonly believe the misconception that traditional chiropractic is habit forming. People tend to think of all healthcare professions in the same way. Within the profession of medicine, there are obviously many pharmaceutical products that are utilized when treating various diseases. Many of these products are dangerous chemicals that are habit forming. Because these chemicals are quite dangerous, drug treatments often require constant supervision by medical specialists.

Chiropractic is a drugless healthcare profession and unlike many traditional medical procedures, there is absolutely nothing addictive about chiropractic care. Patients that visit chiropractors, to get their spines checked for vertebral subluxations, often choose to maintain a long term professional relationship with their doctors. Chiropractic is a preventive healthcare practice, and when patients learn about the many benefits that are associated with being under the care of a chiropractor, it is not uncommon for these individuals to maintain a regular program of lifetime care.

A patient's decision to routinely remain under chiropractic care is often perceived by others in the community as something that is addictive. Hence, the stereotypical habit forming label is often unfairly placed on the chiropractic profession.

Can I go to a Chiropractor if I'm Pregnant?

When a woman becomes pregnant, it is very common for medical doctors to treat her as if she had a disease. Allopathic practitioners regularly attach a diagnosis code in the patient's chart and proceed to treat the condition of pregnancy as a sickness. Insurance products obviously cover the condition of pregnancy and so there are naturally many procedures and medical protocols that are billed to a patient over a nine month period of time.

Just about any other animal on our planet is capable of delivering its offspring in a natural environment without a group of medical specialists standing around a birthing table. Some animals routinely birth an entire litter of offspring at the same time without any complications. A horse, cow, giraffe and countless other examples could be cited to demonstrate that the birthing process is not a disease but rather a natural process within nature that has been artificially complicated by traditional medicine when it comes to human beings.

If it makes good sense to get your spine checked for vertebral subluxations when you are not pregnant, it would logically make good sense to get your spine checked when you are pregnant. It is perfectly safe for women to receive chiropractic adjustments during their entire pregnancy.

There are many ways to modify adjusting techniques through the various stages of a woman's pregnancy, and women should take full advantage of getting under chiropractic care during pregnancy.

Ideally, you always want your body functioning at its full potential. In the case of pregnancy, when a child is forming and growing, it is especially important for a woman's body to be operating as efficiently as possible.

How Often Should I Visit a Chiropractor?

It is a common practice for most people to visit a healthcare professional when they become sick. In reality, most healthcare professionals are actually sickness care specialists and not healthcare professionals because they do not see their patients when they are healthy. Allopathic practitioners specialize in treating people who are suffering from ailments and not individuals that are looking to maintain a state of optimal health.

Doctors of chiropractic are true healthcare specialists because they routinely see their patients when they are feeling well and not exhibiting symptoms or active disease processes. One of the most difficult concepts for laypersons to grasp is the fact that many chiropractic patients regularly visit their chiropractors when they are feeling absolutely fine.

Subluxations that can occur in the human spine, for the most part, do not cause noticeable symptoms or discomfort. Patients cannot always tell if they have one or more subluxated vertebrae in their spines unless they get checked by a qualified chiropractor.

The frequency of chiropractic care is different for each patient. Every person's spine is unique and so therefore it is not practical to make a general recommendation about how often someone should see his or her chiropractor. Usually, the frequency of visits for a chiropractic program is determined by how long a patient is able to maintain adequate spinal alignment. Depending on muscle imbalances within the patient's spinal column, degenerative changes to the vertebrae and of course a lot of other factors, the frequency of care could vary between a couple of visits per week to a couple of visits every few months.

The frequency of care for a patient is always based on objective chiropractic findings that are derived from analytical protocols that have been designed to measure the integrity of spinal alignment. The traditional chiropractor never determines the frequency of chiropractic care based on the presence or absence of symptoms that patients may or may not be reporting.

Health Insurance and Chiropractic

Most health insurance plans do not cover traditional, wellness based, chiropractic care. Any health insurance policies that cover chiropractic visits usually do so on a limited basis. The eligible coverage is usually limited to what is commonly defined as *"crisis"* or *"corrective"* chiropractic care. Most health insurance policies have very strict guidelines that clearly point out the exclusions and limitations associated with reimbursing policyholders for chiropractic visits.

Because the health insurance issue is a complicated subject, I thought that it would be prudent to offer readers a concise and simple explanation about what is usually not covered by health insurance plans in a chiropractor's office and more important, why!

Traditional chiropractic care that is defined as "maintenance" or "wellness" in nature is usually excluded from health insurance reimbursement. These exclusions are also applicable to the federal government's Medicare and Medicaid programs.

The professional care that most traditional chiropractors offer is *"wellness based"* and usually not eligible for insurance reimbursement. Traditional chiropractors do not diagnose specific medical conditions, nor do they issue insurance diagnostic codes on itemized bills that would attempt to suggest a specific condition should be considered for insurance reimbursement.

Most traditional chiropractors set their professional fees in a manner that is consistent with asking patients to utilize wellness based services on a regular basis. In addition, most traditional practitioners offer professional fees that are both affordable and fair for all members of the community.

In most traditional chiropractic practices, the patients must consider how valuable the care they are receiving is and also if they want "for profit" insurance companies to determine whether they should continue to receive future care.

Unfortunately, most chiropractic patients terminate their professional relationships with a specific practitioner once their insurance benefits have been exhausted. This leaves many patients without adequate chiropractic care throughout the year. It also leaves patients with a poor understanding of how regular chiropractic care can benefit all human beings.

What's wrong with this Picture?

It's not very easy to convince people that a vertebral subluxation is a serious problem. In fact, I believe that convincing healthcare consumers that a subluxation can cause devastating effects to the human body is one of the most daunting tasks in the world. The average person has never heard of this condition and is unaware of the damage a subluxation can do to human physiology.

Certain conditions of sickness, which a large portion of society seem to be concerned about, have been prominently advertised via the mainstream media. The various diseases that are in the forefront of people's minds today (cancer, rheumatoid arthritis, lupus, diabetes, etc.) have support groups, fund raisers, parades, walkathons, and other elements of fanfare attached to them. These are the types of publicity campaigns that are necessary in order to create a high degree of public awareness about a particular health condition.

As I have written earlier in this book, very large and powerful pharmaceutical corporations have the unlimited resources necessary to create awareness about specific conditions – and they do! The health conditions which are regularly discussed on the evening news or featured in popular magazines and on Internet websites have been big money producers for the pharmaceutical companies for many years. The drug products sold to manage these illnesses are extremely expensive and, in the case of autoimmune diseases, the drugs are also extremely dangerous as they create their intended effect by shutting down the body's immune system functions.

In the treatment of cancer, all drugs currently being used are experimental in nature because there are no cures available. The treatments are all very much based on inhibition of the body's natural physiology in an attempt to modify or alleviate a patient's symptoms. In looking at this dilemma from a physiological perspective, it is not a stretch to write that modern medicine will never cure a single disease process based on the type of research that is being performed.

All the double blind studies in the world, with sophisticated laboratory settings, will never produce a cure for a single disease because the general focus of such research is centered on managing and controlling the effects of diseases. There is not much research, if any, being performed to address the cause of diseases. There's also no great desire, by the Medical Establishment, to eradicate any of the lucrative disorders in question.

Another Double Blind Study Looking For...

...The Answer to Cancer!

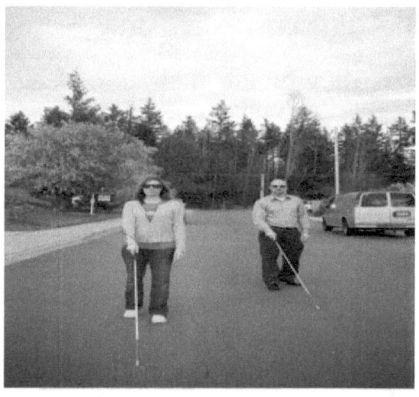

Figure 11 - © Mat Hayward - Fotolia.com

If you think that my statement about modern medicine never finding a cure for any disease whatsoever is silly, just take a few moments to think about how long scientists have been performing medical research. They've been at this task for many years and the results of their work have produced no cures to date. The research being performed is not searching for cures and so none will be found.

The very sad thing about the entire medical situation is that the profession has a batting average of zero when it comes to curing the human body of any diseases. Yet the Medical Establishment, and the cronies that work for them, keep telling the world that the profession of medicine is very scientific. What is being held out and marketed to the world as *the best science has to offer,* is yielding worse than awful results. In keeping with the baseball analogy, even a major league pitcher who doesn't spend a lot of time in the batting cage, sticks out the bat and gets a lucky hit once in a while.

The chiropractic debunkers keep screaming about how much science is behind medical research and that chiropractic is not valid because some double blind studies haven't been performed. In my opinion, all that science backing the medical profession's disease management programs doesn't seem to be working out too well for the patients suffering with various diseases.

If the mainstream media campaigns could be used to teach healthcare consumers about the dangers associated with vertebral subluxation and the importance of getting a spinal examination by a competent chiropractor, the world would be filled with a lot of healthy people.

In an alternative version of reality, the evening news would talk about natural health concepts and the commercials wouldn't feature actors smiling as they attempted to convince healthcare consumers to take various poisons. In that world there would be walkathons to raise awareness about vertebral subluxation and news articles in major magazines that discussed the importance of having all children examined by a chiropractor instead of receiving toxic vaccines.

In this alternative version of reality, a lot of drug companies would lose billions of dollars and the stock market would probably tank, but that's a small price for society to pay in order to assure its citizens better health.

The profit that a pharmaceutical company makes in a year is several hundred million dollars. The profit that the entire Medical Establishment makes in the same amount of time is in the billions of dollars. The cost to research countless numbers of drugs, utilizing double blind studies, is mind boggling. The results that the research will yield are zero cures.

The price tag to research the effectiveness of a chiropractic adjustment being administered to a human spine that is subluxated would be zero dollars. The research was already performed by B.J. Palmer, the developer of chiropractic many years ago. Chiropractic worked then and it still works today! The price tag to ensure that every child, man and woman in our country received a chiropractic examination and adjustment if necessary would be nominal, but the results would be absolutely—priceless!

Tying Everything Together

Several years ago I wrote a short story that highlighted the contrasting paradigms tied to traditional chiropractic and modern allopathic medicine. I really think the story sums up the concepts I have written about in this book and I wanted to include it here for readers. Enjoy!

"The Town of Sickville"

Once upon a time, there was a small town named Sickville. Sickville was an economically thriving community and its entire financial well being was dependent on a number of health care companies that regularly provided services to the many citizens living within its borders.

According to the local census bureau, Sickville had a population of 2000. Approximately 450 of the townspeople were health care practitioners. The remainder of the residents worked in other health related occupations.

Many of Sickville's citizens were staff members at one of six local hospitals. Others drove the 25 delivery trucks that routinely carried medical supplies to 35 community drugstores. The remainder of the population worked for the locally owned ambulance company. The small town proudly operated 50, state-of-the-art, patient transport vehicles.

Almost every resident of Sickville earned a good living. Ninety-eight percent of the population had no mortgage or car payments. The people of Sickville seemed to have plenty of money to buy whatever they wanted, and many of them had become wealthy.

Unfortunately, most of Sickville's population was not very healthy. The citizens couldn't enjoy the money they were earning. People were often too sick to go on vacations and take part in other fun activities. Most of the townspeople were challenged with chronic colds and recurring bouts of influenza. Others suffered with autoimmune disorders, cardiovascular disease and diabetes. A growing number of citizens had recently developed more serious illnesses, like cancer and leukemia.

Very few of the town's residents had all of their body parts. In Sickville it was considered a normal practice to have elective surgery for precautionary measures. Useless organs, that often caused problems later in a person's life like gallbladders, appendices, and tonsils, were routinely removed by one of the town's 56 surgeons. Men and women were also regularly encouraged to have vasectomies and hysterectomies after the age of 45. These were *common sense health practices,* routinely taught and reinforced in the Sickville Public School system.

A very small number of individuals, living in Sickville (about 25), were homeless people. They were the ones that didn't have an official disease yet; but it was only a matter of time before they would be diagnosed with one. Every resident living in Sickville became unhealthy sooner or later. That's why there was always such a big demand for medical doctors and other health care services.

The townspeople referred to the homeless people as *the poor and unfortunate ones* that roamed around looking for handouts. None of them could afford quality health care services, so they missed out on the disease prevention programs that the more affluent citizens regularly took advantage of.

A new town ordinance had recently been passed requiring every citizen living in Sickville to visit a medical physician at least once per week. The regular medical visits ensured all residents, except for the homeless people, were up-to-date on vaccines and other preventive healthcare protocols that had been established by the local medical board.

Preventive care was a big deal in Sickville. The town's medical doctors had determined, many years earlier, the only way to ward off newer and deadlier diseases was to continue to develop and administer an assortment of vaccines. The medical board had declared an all out *war on sickness*.

Another new law required the residents of Sickville to proudly display their diagnosed diseases on the front of their driver's licenses. The local medical board felt it was important for the town council members to keep track of all illnesses that were currently active within the community. This was because officially diagnosed diseases translated into profitable revenue streams for the entire town.

One September afternoon, something very unusual happened in Sickville. A new doctor moved into the only vacant building in town. This practitioner was different from other doctors. He prescribed no medicines;

administered no vaccines; performed no surgeries, and didn't wear a white coat. He called himself a chiropractor.

Quickly, the chiropractor opened his professional office inside the once vacant building. The people of Sickville were very curious about the new doctor. He had only brought with him a few chairs for his waiting room and a strange looking table that he used to work on his patients.

At first, the chiropractor only took care of the community's homeless people. He bartered with his patients instead of charging them a fee. In return, the patients painted his office and helped him in other ways. He'd ask his patients to lie on the strange table and would feel their backs. Every once in a while he'd push his hands down, forcefully, onto their spines. That's, pretty much, all the chiropractor would do.

It didn't take very long for gossip to get out to the other people of Sickville. The gossip began traveling fast about how the chiropractor practiced a strange brand of medicine. Many townspeople thought he was crazy – a quack!

After awhile, some of the other citizens in town began going to the chiropractor. They enjoyed visiting him because he taught them interesting concepts they'd never heard before from other healthcare practitioners.

The chiropractor explained to his new patients how the human brain sent important messages to the entire body through the spinal cord and how the spine protected the spinal cord. He also explained how spinal adjustments helped to realign the spinal bones when they became misaligned from one another. The chiropractor told his patients that once the spinal bones were properly aligned, the brain's messages could get through to the entire body and health could be restored naturally, without taking drugs.

The chiropractor also explained that when the nervous system worked properly, and wasn't being interfered with by misaligned spinal bones, the townspeople would be healthier, and they wouldn't have to surgically remove their body parts. He explained that the removal of tonsils, appendices, and gallbladders was not really a smart thing to do. The chiropractor also went on to explain that receiving vaccines was a waste of time and that the shots harmed their immune systems. The chiropractor told the members of the community that many of the harmful diseases the people of Sickville were experiencing were coming from the preventive vaccines and that vaccinations, in general, were preventing good health from being expressed in their bodies.

A year after the chiropractor opened his office; many of the townspeople were visiting him for spinal adjustments on a weekly basis. Hundreds of the residents were now under regular chiropractic care. The new chiropractic patients stopped visiting the other doctors and they stopped buying prescription drugs and getting vaccinations. They also stopped scheduling surgeries to remove their organs.

Because people weren't visiting medical doctors, the physicians began moving out of Sickville to look for work in other nearby communities. The surgeons left too because the townspeople no longer wanted to have their body parts removed.

It didn't take very long for the six hospitals to feel the effects of a decrease in business. All but one of the facilities had to close its doors. The one hospital that remained open had a lot of vacant space and decided to rent the empty parts of the building to the new chiropractor. He opened a satellite office and hired 2 additional chiropractors to help take care of all the new chiropractic patients.

Plenty of people in Sickville were beginning to get well. Almost all the diseases the townspeople had experienced, for so many years, had miraculously disappeared.

Unfortunately, as luck would have it, the community of Sickville began to experience financially hard times. A recession had mysteriously hit the entire area. It soon turned into an economic depression. The town was only able to keep one ambulance operating, and 33 of the 35 drugstores had to close due to low sales. Financially speaking, it was a terrible time.

At one point the economy got so bad that quite a few townspeople lost their jobs. Many residents were forced to take out mortgages on their homes in order to pay for living expenses. After awhile, residents couldn't make their mortgage payments and lost homes to foreclosure. The previously wealthy citizens of Sickville were broke and forced to live in shelters with the other homeless people.

One night, the local members of the medical board got together and held a secret meeting. They discussed, at length, the town's unhealthy economy. They blamed the community's financial problems on the new chiropractor that had moved into town. They concluded it was his radical and unscientific ideas that had destroyed most of the health care businesses in Sickville.

The medical board conducted a vote and unanimously decided to outlaw the practice of chiropractic in Sickville. They rationalized that the practice of chiropractic was based on pseudoscience and was a direct threat to the health and well being of all citizens. In one secret meeting, the medical board had solved the town's biggest problem.

The very next day, the chiropractor cleared out his office and left Sickville. The townspeople were upset at first, but they soon forgot about the strange doctor with the funny table that pressed on backs.

A new practitioner immediately moved into the chiropractor's vacant office. He was a real doctor that prescribed drugs; performed surgeries; administered vaccines, and most important, wore a white coat.

Within a few months, people started getting sick all over again. Soon after that, the medical doctors returned to town. Even the surgeons came back to Sickville. People were losing their health rapidly and desperately needed to have useless organs removed. The hospital system seemed to expand overnight. Inside of a year, the six hospitals were back in business and filled to capacity. There was even talk about building a seventh hospital.

The ambulance company was busy again, too, just like old times. They managed to increase their fleet of patient transport vehicles to 53. People were sicker than ever. In fact, there were so many different epidemics taking place at the same time, the medical board decided to purchase three times the normal amount of vaccines for the hospitals and drugstores.

Sickville had definitely returned to the way it was before the strange doctor, who pressed on backs, had come to town. People were so ill; they were dying faster than any other time in the town's recorded history.

The only consolation for the Sickville townspeople was that the economy had finally begun to recover. Because the citizens were so ill, they had generated revenue streams like never before. Almost every citizen managed to climb out of debt. Money was changing hands like crazy and the residents of Sickville were able to buy back their homes and purchase new cars. The depression was officially over and the economy was healthier than ever. Too bad nobody could enjoy the money they were earning.

Afterword

As people, we make choices in life that directly or indirectly affect our abilities to remain healthy. In other words, our physiology is continuously challenged by the foods, poisons and environmental conditions we encounter.

The physiological construct of any living organism is quite complex. Obviously, some organisms are more complex in their design than others. Regardless of the complexity of various forms of life, it's important to realize that all living things share a commonality of innate intelligence. All living organisms have an inner wisdom that strives to maintain their existence in our world. Without this innate logic, living organisms would not be capable of surviving for very long.

In human beings, the inborn intelligence I write about is constantly expressed in the body through the nervous system. This vital lifeline is the conduit that allows or disallows health to be present throughout our lives.

It is my belief that chiropractic is a very safe and affordable vehicle for healthcare consumers to utilize in an effort to achieve and maintain a better expression of health during the course of their lives.

I hope that you have enjoyed reading this material as much as I have enjoyed writing it. The explanations in this book about how traditional chiropractic works as well as how the Medical Establishment attacks the profession and its practitioners, need to be read by everyone that has a desire to be healthy.

Throughout this book, I have attempted to provide readers with pertinent information, analogies and general knowledge about health that I have acquired throughout my professional career as a practicing chiropractor. I genuinely hope that my writings will help persuade people to consider visiting a chiropractor for wellness based care in the near future.

-Dr. John Reizer

Suggested Reading:

BOOKS:

"Natural Alternative to Vaccination (Natural Health Guide)"
by Zoltan P. Rona

"Confessions of a Medical Heretic"
by Robert S. Mendelsohn

"A Shot in the Dark"
by Harris L. Coulter

"Vaccination: State Sponsored Murder"
by M.P., Arnold Lupton

"The Poisoned Needle: Suppressed Facts about Vaccination"
by Eleanor McBean

"Vaccination Horror: An Anthology of Important Works on Vaccination Pseudoscience" by John Drake

"The Vaccination Myth: Courageous MD Exposes the Vaccination Fraud!"
by Charles Creighton, M.D.

WEBSITES:

www.mercola.com
http://educate-yourself.org/vcd/
www.thinktwice.com
www.tetrahedron.org/